PLANT BASED MEDICINE

A Complete Guide For Addressing Challenges And Unraveling The Secrets Of Herbal Preparations And Formulations For Holistic Wellness

WALTER ZYAIRE

DISCLAIMER

The information in this book is intended only for general informational purposes; it should not be used in lieu of professional advice or medical care. Since the author is not licensed to practice therapy, the information offered should not be used in place of the expertise, judgment, or guidance of qualified mental health or medical professionals. Readers are encouraged to consult therapists, medical specialists, or other qualified authorities regarding their particular situation and needs. The publisher and author disclaim all liability for any actions or decisions taken by readers based on the information in this book. Results may vary from person to person and this book's approaches, procedures, and strategies may not be suitable in all circumstances. Considering unique situations and consulting a qualified expert are essential when choosing the right course of action. Neither the publisher nor the author recommend or guarantee the efficacy of any therapy or treatment that is indicated in this book. Because the information is based on the author's research and understanding at the time of publishing, it could not reflect the most recent developments or practices in the treatment area. The publisher and the author both disclaim all liability for the accuracy, completeness, or use of the material in this book. Readers bear full responsibility for the decisions and actions they choose in light of the information presented in this book.

TABLE OF CONTENTS

ABOUT THE BOOK

"Plant-Based Medicine: A Comprehensive Guide" is an essential tool for anyone looking to learn more about the significant effects of plant-based therapy on human health. The book starts with a thoughtful introduction that lays out its goals and highlights the significance of plant-based medicine in the current healthcare environment.

The definition of plant-based medicine and its historical background are explored, providing insight into its customary uses in medical procedures. To promote overall well-being, the book emphasizes the value of adopting plant-based healing techniques. The scientific foundations of plant-based medicine are then examined, which also clarifies the functions of phytochemicals and looks at the complex interactions between plants and the human body. The abundance of studies and research demonstrating the effectiveness of plant-based healing is also highlighted in this section.

Readers are given useful information on assembling an herbal medicine kit. It lists plants that should be in every beginner's kit, offers advice on gathering and preserving medicinal herbs, and shows how to make tinctures, infusions, and extracts. The book goes on to discuss common illnesses and associated plant-based treatments, providing workable answers for problems like headaches, stomachaches, tension, anxiety, and sleep disturbances.

The topic of bringing plant medicine into daily life is covered. Some techniques that are suggested are using natural skincare and beauty recipes, making herbal teas and infusions, and cooking with medicinal plants. The next few chapters focus on specific subjects, on plant medicine for women's health and on plant-based family and children's medicine.

The book delves into ethical aspects by examining sustainable methods in plant medicine, ethical sourcing of plant-based goods, and responsible foraging and cultivation.

The future of plant-based medicine is explored. Research advancements, integrative healthcare approaches, and future problems and opportunities are highlighted.

"Plant-Based Medicine: A Comprehensive Guide" is an invaluable tool that encourages readers to embrace the therapeutic potential of plants in their daily lives in addition to imparting knowledge. For those looking for a holistic approach to well-being, herbal lovers, and healthcare professionals alike, this extensive resource is a must-have.

CHAPTER ONE

OVERVIEW OF PLANT-BASED MEDICINE

PLANT-BASED MEDICINE'S PLACE IN HEALTHCARE

The promise of plant-based medicine to promote holistic well-being has drawn increased interest in the ever-evolving field of healthcare. Plant-based medicine, sometimes referred to as herbal medicine or phytotherapy is the application of compounds obtained from plants for medicinal purposes.

This age-old method of healing has a long history and is ingrained in many different cultures around the globe. Gaining knowledge about the foundations, background, and importance of plant-based medicine can help you better understand how it fits into modern healthcare procedures.

COMPREHENDING PLANT-BASED MEDICINE

Fundamentally, plant-based therapy works by using the medicinal qualities of different plant parts, like leaves, roots, flowers, and seeds, to treat a wide range of illnesses. Plant-based medicine has its historical origins in ancient civilizations when indigenous groups learned about the therapeutic benefits of plants via trial and error and passed on this traditional knowledge to succeeding generations. The variety of plant-based treatments found in different cultures demonstrates how widely held the notion that nature can heal is.

MEANING AND BACKGROUND

Plant-based medicine is more than just herbal remedies; it's a comprehensive approach that recognizes the body, mind, and environment as being interdependent. This paradigm places a strong emphasis on treating illnesses from the inside out as opposed to only treating their symptoms. The complex biological systems of the human body and the synergistic effects of active substances within them are just two aspects of the diverse nature of plant-based treatment.

THE VALUE OF PLANT-BASED REMEDIES

The growing understanding of the drawbacks and adverse effects of synthetic medications highlights the significance of plant-based healing in modern healthcare. There is an increasing interest in investigating complementary and alternative medicine in addition to conventional medicine as communities struggle with problems like antibiotic resistance and harmful drug reactions. With its focus on natural substances, plant-based medicine is a viable option for treating medical issues while reducing adverse effects on patients and the environment.

CUSTOMARY APPLICATIONS OF PLANTS IN MEDICINE

For many generations, traditional medical techniques have used plants, and for many communities, this has been the main source of treatment. Indigenous knowledge systems have long acknowledged the therapeutic potential of plants and have used them to cure a broad range of illnesses, from chronic illnesses to infectious infections. This conventional wisdom stresses the cultural importance and spiritual ties that frequently go along with plant-based therapeutic methods in addition to the effectiveness of these treatments.

Research into plant-based medicine reveals a complex picture braided with historical relevance, holistic ideas, and the possibility of a more peaceful and sustainable method of treating patients. We learn more about the potential advantages that this age-old but ongoing practice provides for the well-being of both individuals and communities as we explore the various traditions that have embraced plant-based healing.

CHAPTER TWO

THE SCIENTIFIC BASIS OF PLANT-BASED THERAPEUTICS

PHYTOCHEMICALS: THEIR FUNCTIONS

Plants contain bioactive substances called phytochemicals, sometimes referred to as phytonutrients, which help explain some of their therapeutic qualities. These chemical substances are essential to the health advantages of plant-based medicine. Phytochemicals are produced by plants for a variety of uses, such as defense against microbe infections, environmental stresses, and predators. Phytochemicals have anti-inflammatory, antioxidant, and anti-cancer properties within the human body. Flavonoids, alkaloids, terpenoids, and polyphenols are a few types of phytochemicals. Each has certain qualities that enhance the therapeutic potential of medications derived from plants.

THE HUMAN BODY'S INTERACTION WITH PLANTS

The human body and plants interact through intricate processes that are yet poorly understood. Enzymes in the digestive system break down plant substances into smaller molecules for simpler assimilation, which is where phytochemical absorption starts. After being ingested, these phytochemicals can have an impact on cellular functions and enhance health through interactions with different biological pathways.

Certain phytochemicals, for example, have the same effects as human hormones, while others may prevent the formation of aberrant cells. The complex interactions that occur between plant-based chemicals and the human body highlight how varied and multidimensional plant-based therapy is.

STUDIES AND RESEARCH ON PLANT-BASED HEALING

Recent years have seen a major increase in the amount of research and studies on plant-based healing, which has helped to clarify the workings and effectiveness of many treatments derived from plants. Research studies examine the possibility of using plant-based substances to treat a variety of illnesses, including infectious disorders and chronic illnesses. For instance, research has shown that the antioxidant curcumin from turmeric, the heart-healthy resveratrol from grapes, and the immune-stimulating qualities of echinacea all have anti-inflammatory qualities. To assess the efficacy and safety of plant-based therapies, researchers use a range of approaches, such as observational studies, laboratory experiments, and clinical trials.

More and more research is pointing to the therapeutic potential of plant-based medicine, with findings indicating that in some circumstances, these natural therapies could even take the place of traditional medications. Plant-based healing takes a holistic approach that takes into account the synergistic effects of several components inside a plant in addition to the separated substances. Furthermore, researching traditional medical practices from other cultures offers insightful information on the possible uses of plant-based medicines. A deeper comprehension of the science underlying plant-based medicine is becoming apparent as research in this area progresses, opening the door to creative and long-lasting methods of providing healthcare.

CHAPTER THREE

PUTTING TOGETHER YOUR HERBAL MEDICINE KIT

CRUCIAL PLANTS FOR A KIT FOR BEGINNERS

Choosing essential plants with a range of therapeutic uses is the first step in assembling a beginner's herbal medicine kit. Because of its relaxing and anti-inflammatory properties, chamomile is a well-liked option among the important herbs. It is frequently used to treat stomach problems and stress. Renowned for its ability to strengthen the immune system, echinacea is another important component of the kit. This plant can be especially helpful during the cold and flu seasons since it aids the body in fighting off infections. Lavender is a great addition to encouraging relaxation and supporting sleep because of its calming scent and moderate sedative qualities.

Furthermore, peppermint is a multipurpose herb well-known for helping with digestion and relieving headaches. Its leaves can be the foundation for infusions or added to teas. Calendula is beneficial for skin health and wound healing because of its antibacterial and anti-inflammatory qualities. Finally, elderberry is a powerful immune-boosting herb that is frequently used in tinctures or syrups to treat the flu and cold.

GATHERING AND PRESERVING HERBAL REMEDIES

It's important to comprehend the life cycle of the plant and the best seasons to harvest therapeutic plants. When flowers or leaves are in full bloom, a plant's medicinal effectiveness is at its highest, thus it's important to harvest it then.

To preserve the essential oils in the plant, harvesting should be done early in the morning after the dew has dried but before the sun rises. Plant damage is reduced and a more efficient harvest is guaranteed when clean, sharp tools are used.

Preserving the medicinal properties of the plants requires careful drying and storage. Herbs are typically dried by air, although other methods, including using a dehydrator or hanging bundles upside down, may work better for specific plants. To avoid moisture and light deterioration, keep dried herbs in airtight containers in a cold, dark spot.

MAKING EXTRACTS, INFUSIONS, AND TINCTURES

Making tinctures, infusions, and extracts is the process of transforming gathered plants into useful products. Herbal remedies can be efficiently preserved and concentrated with tinctures, which are extracts made with alcohol. The procedure calls for soaking the herb for many weeks in high-proof alcohol, such as vodka or brandy, then stirring the mixture frequently to aid in extraction.

Conversely, infusions entail steeping plants in hot water to draw out their therapeutic properties.

This technique is frequently applied to fragile herbs, such as peppermint or chamomile. Infusions can be used topically for a variety of uses or drunk as teas.

Herbal medication in concentrated form is called an extract, which is frequently made with a mixture of alcohol and water. They are strong and usually need expert assistance to prepare properly. By making these diverse herbal concoctions, novices can experiment with the many uses of therapeutic herbs, meeting personal tastes and medical requirements.

CHAPTER FOUR

COMMON ILLNESSES AND HERBAL TREATMENTS

MIGRAINES & HEADACHES

Common conditions like headaches and migraines can have a big influence on day-to-day activities. Although over-the-counter drugs are frequently utilized to treat symptoms, plant-based therapies can provide more natural options. For example, the herb feverfew is well-known for its ability to lessen migraine frequency and intensity. Because of its anti-inflammatory qualities, it might make headache pain less severe.

Furthermore, applying peppermint oil topically to the temples has been shown to have a calming effect, providing relief from tension headaches. Because ginger reduces nausea and inflammation, including it in the diet may also help prevent migraines.

PROBLEMS WITH THE DIGESTIVE SYSTEM

Irritable bowel syndrome (IBS), bloating, and indigestion are just a few of the illnesses that fall under the category of digestive difficulties. Using plant-based therapies can be very important for supporting digestive health. For instance, peppermint tea is well known for its capacity to ease indigestion and bloating by relaxing the muscles of the digestive system. Because of its anti-inflammatory qualities, ginger may help with IBS symptoms. Fermented foods, such as kimchi and sauerkraut, include probiotics that support healthy gut flora and facilitate nutrient absorption and digestion.

ANXIETY AND STRESS

Anxiety and stress are common issues in the fast-paced world of today. Plant-based therapies provide a comprehensive strategy for handling these problems. Herbs that are known to assist the body adapt to stressors, such as Rhodiola and ashwagandha, have long been used to support a balanced reaction to anxiety-inducing circumstances. By utilizing teas or essential oils, one can naturally soothe the mind and reduce tension by utilizing the relaxing effects of chamomile and lavender. Herbal medicines and mindfulness exercises can be used in a comprehensive stress and anxiety management plan.

DISORDERS OF SLEEP

Although getting enough sleep is crucial for general health, sleep disorders are becoming more prevalent. Plant-based therapies have the potential to improve sleep quality. For generations, people have utilized the calming qualities of Valerian root to enhance the quality of their sleep. Because of its relaxing properties, passionflower may aid in lowering insomnia and enhancing sleep habits. Furthermore, the practice of indulging in warm herbal teas, such as valerian or chamomile, before bedtime might help the body relax and promote a more seamless sleeps transition. Including these plant-based medicines in a soothing nighttime routine will help you get a better night's sleep.

BOOSTERS OF THE IMMUNE SYSTEM

Keeping the immune system strong is essential to avoiding diseases. A range of minerals and chemicals that enhance immune function can be found in plant-based therapies. Elderberries are said to strengthen the immune system and shorten the duration of colds and the flu because they are high in antioxidants and vitamins. Echinacea has long been utilized as an immune system stimulant and a potential defense against respiratory infections. Including immune-stimulating herbs in meals, such as turmeric and garlic, offers even more assistance. A varied range of nutrients necessary for general immunological health is ensured by a plant-based diet that is well-balanced and abundant in fruits, vegetables, and whole grains.

CHAPTER FIVE

INCLUDING PLANT MEDICINE IN EVERYDAY ACTIVITIES

USING THERAPEUTIC PLANTS IN COOKING

Using medicinal herbs in everyday life requires a comprehensive strategy that goes beyond their conventional medical application. Cooking is one easy approach to include plant-based healing qualities. A wide variety of medicinal plants can be explored by foodies and health-conscious people alike since they enhance flavor and promote general well-being in meals.

For example, adding herbs such as rosemary, thyme, and basil to food improves its flavor while also adding healthful components that have antioxidant and anti-inflammatory qualities. People can make everyday meals into nourishing experiences by intentionally choosing their herbs and spices.

HERBAL INFUSIONS AND TEAS

Herbal infusions and teas provide an additional way to incorporate plant medicine into everyday life. Herbal teas offer a chance to tap into the restorative properties of plants in addition to their cozy warmth and calming fragrances. Ginger, peppermint, and chamomile are a few examples of the varieties that have long been prized for their therapeutic qualities, which include stress reduction and digestive support.

These teas can be customized to meet the specific needs of each person by adding other therapeutic herbs, such as lemon balm or echinacea, to the blend. Frequent ingestion of these teas facilitates a more profound connection with the restorative qualities of nature, in addition to being a joyful ritual.

NATURAL BEAUTY AND SKINCARE RECIPES

A third way to incorporate plant medicine into daily life is through natural skincare and cosmetic recipes.

An increasing number of people in the beauty business are interested in using medicinal herbs for skincare. Calendula, aloe vera, and lavender are among the ingredients that are well-known for their calming and nourishing properties on the skin.

These natural substances can be used by individuals to make their skincare products, such as moisturizers, toners, and face masks. This method not only encourages healthier skin but also lessens dependency on manufactured goods that contain artificial chemicals. Adopting natural skincare practices encourages a deliberate and attentive relationship with the medicinal properties of plants.

Using medicinal plants in everyday life entails more than just using them to treat particular illnesses. People can incorporate the healing properties of plants into their everyday routines by using them in their food, herbal teas, and cosmetics regimens.

CHAPTER SIX

USING PLANT MEDICINE

HORMONAL BALANCE AND WOMEN'S HEALTH

For millennia, women have been helped to achieve hormonal balance through the use of plant medicine. Many herbs and botanicals have adaptogenic qualities, which support the body's ability to adjust to stimuli and preserve hormonal balance. Adaptogens, which include holy basil and ashwagandha, are well-known for their capacity to uplift the endocrine system and assist in the control of hormones like estrogen and cortisol. Furthermore, plants high in phytoestrogens, such as flaxseed and red clover, may offer a safe and gentle method of regulating estrogen levels, promoting hormonal balance overall.

MENSTRUAL PROBLEMS

Plant-based therapies are an important part of treating menstrual problems since they give women options besides traditional medications. Premenstrual syndrome (PMS) symptoms have historically been treated with herbs like chaste tree (Vitex agnus-castus), which work by altering the balance of reproductive hormones.

Moreover, the anti-inflammatory qualities of ginger and turmeric may help lessen the pain and suffering associated with menstruation. Moreover, raspberry leaf tea has gained popularity due to its ability to strengthen the uterine muscles, which may lessen the discomfort associated with menstrual cramps.

ASSISTANCE DURING PREGNANCY AND POSTPARTUM

Plant medicine is a useful tool for women going through these stages since it offers the mother and the growing fetus natural assistance. Nettle leaf is frequently advised to meet nutritional demands during pregnancy because it is rich in important elements like calcium and iron.

Red raspberry leaf is well known for its uterine toning properties, which may facilitate a more seamless birth. Furthermore, during the taxing postpartum phase, the adaptogenic qualities of herbs like ashwagandha and astragalus may help with stress management and general well-being promotion.

Herbs like blessed thistle and fenugreek are frequently used to help nursing moms boost lactation throughout the postpartum period. It is said that these herbs increase milk production and offer extra nutritional advantages to the nursing child and mother.

Herbs that are known to be calming, such as lemon balm and chamomile, can also help reduce tension and anxiety, which will support emotional health during the difficult postpartum phase.

A holistic and natural approach to well-being is reflected in the use of plant medicine in women's health, particularly in resolving menstrual difficulties, preserving hormonal balance, and offering pregnancy and postpartum care.

A compassionate and efficient way to support a woman at different stages of her reproductive journey is to incorporate these herbal treatments into women's healthcare practices.

CHAPTER SEVEN

PLANT-BASED TREATMENT FOR FAMILIES AND CHILDREN

KID-FRIENDLY SOLUTIONS

It is important to give priority to child-friendly medicines that are not only effective but also tasty and simple to administer while researching plant-based medicine for families and children. For example, herbal teas can be a gentle yet effective treatment for common childhood illnesses. Because of its calming qualities, chamomile tea can help ease digestive problems or encourage relaxation before bed.

Likewise, youngsters experiencing mild respiratory pain may get relief from the symptoms with peppermint tea. Other kid-friendly medicines that are simple to add to a child's routine are tinctures and syrups derived from herbs like licorice root, elderberry, and echinacea.

INCREASING THE IMMUNE SYSTEMS OF CHILDREN

Improving kids' immune systems is essential to supporting their general health. There are several natural ways to boost and fortify the immune system with plant-based medicines. Nutrient-dense foods and herbal supplements can be used to include a range of immune-boosting herbs in children's diets. For instance, elderberry is well known for boosting the immune system and comes in a variety of kid-friendly forms, such as syrups and candies. Furthermore, adding turmeric, ginger, and garlic to food boosts immunity in addition to adding flavor. The long-term maintenance of a healthy immune system in children requires providing them with a diet rich in plants and balanced.

SAFETY OBSERVATIONS

Plant-based medication has the potential to improve children's health, but it must be used carefully and with safety in mind.

It is advised to speak with a medical practitioner before incorporating any new plant-based medicines into a child's daily routine, especially if that individual specializes in pediatric care.

Dosage is a crucial component, and to avoid any negative effects, it is crucial to closely follow the suggested parameters. It is important to seek professional counsel as certain herbs may have contraindications or interact negatively with drugs. To guarantee the quality and purity of herbal goods, it is also crucial to select reliable suppliers. When giving new plant-based medicines to their children, parents should also watch out for potential negative consequences or allergic responses.

Adopting plant-based medicine for kids and families entails taking into account kid-friendly treatments that are simple to use and effective. Encouraging children's immune systems with a plant-based, well-balanced diet and well-chosen herbal supplements can help improve their general health.

To guarantee a safe and happy experience with plant-based treatments for kids, safety concerns should always come first, requiring consultation with medical specialists and following suggested guidelines.

CHAPTER EIGHT

SUSTAINABLE DEVELOPMENT AND ETHICAL HARVESTING

ECO-FRIENDLY METHODS IN PLANT MEDICINE

Sustainable methods are critical to the long-term health and viability of plant populations in the field of plant medicine. This entails using farming techniques that limit harm to the environment and enhance biodiversity. In plant medicine, sustainable techniques cover the full plant lifetime, from growing to harvest, not just the extraction of therapeutic ingredients.

Using agroecological techniques like regenerative farming or permaculture promotes a positive interaction between the production of plant medicines and the ecosystems providing them. This benefits the environment's general health in addition to preserving the purity of the therapeutic plants.

CONSCIENTIOUS GATHERING AND PLANTING

In the field of plant medicine, ethical harvesting involves both responsible farming and foraging. Cultivators and foragers are essential to preserving the delicate equilibrium between ecological preservation and human use. A thorough knowledge of the distinct plant populations, their life cycles, and the environments in which they flourish is necessary for responsible foraging. Organic and sustainable cultivation techniques should take precedence over the use of dangerous pesticides and artificial fertilizers. Crop rotation is another technique that can be used to reduce soil erosion and improve the land's long-term fertility.

ETHICALLY PURCHASING PLANT-BASED GOODS

Plant-based product ethical sourcing is a complex idea that takes social, economic, and environmental factors into account. Fair labor practices, open supplier chains, and an equitable sharing of financial gains throughout the production process are all part of it. Ethical sourcing guarantees that local communities profit from the extraction or development of medicinal plants by addressing issues like community involvement. It also advocates for a prudent method of wild harvesting, making sure that foraging operations do not endanger plant species' survival or devastate the environments in which they are found. To indicate adherence to ethical sourcing norms, certification programs, and labels—such as Fair Trade or Organic—are frequently used. This gives customers the power to choose decisions that are consistent with their values.

Ethical harvesting and sustainability of herbal resources are facilitated by sustainable practices in plant medicine, ethical procurement of plant-based goods, and responsible foraging and cultivation. Adhering to these guidelines guarantees that future generations will be able to make use of the therapeutic qualities of plants, as well as the delicate balance that must be maintained between human use and environmental preservation.

CHAPTER NINE

PLANT-BASED MEDICINE'S FUTURE

PROGRESS IN THE STUDY OF PLANT MEDICINE

Research and development in the field of plant-based medicine have increased significantly in recent years, indicating a growing interest in utilizing the medicinal potential of different plant species. Scientific progress has made it possible to comprehend the chemical components and pharmacological characteristics of plants on a deeper level, which has opened the door to the discovery of new substances with therapeutic uses. This growing body of knowledge has not only made it easier to extract and isolate active ingredients, but it has also accelerated the development of complex plant cultivation methods, guaranteeing a consistent and long-lasting supply for medical use.

Researchers are increasingly researching the complicated links between plants and human health, digging into the synergistic effects of different plant components and their possible applications in treating a wide array of diseases. The identification and isolation of bioactive compounds, such as alkaloids, flavonoids, and terpenoids, have provided a foundation for the synthesis of plant-derived pharmaceuticals with better efficacy and reduced adverse effects. These findings indicate a huge step towards the integration of plant medicine into conventional healthcare, enabling alternative and complementary therapies for many medical ailments.

INTEGRATIVE APPROACHES TO HEALTHCARE

The future of plant-based medicine lies not only in the isolation of individual compounds but also in the integration of these botanical remedies into comprehensive healthcare approaches. The paradigm shift towards integrative medicine emphasizes the combined use of conventional medical treatments with alternative therapies, including plant-based interventions. This holistic approach recognizes the interconnectedness of physical, mental, and emotional well-being, seeking to address the root causes of illness rather than merely alleviating symptoms.

Integrative healthcare models incorporate plant-based medicine into patient-centered treatment plans, considering individual variations in genetics, lifestyle, and environmental factors. The synergy between conventional medicine and plant-based therapies holds the promise of personalized and more effective healthcare solutions. Collaborative efforts between healthcare professionals, herbalists, and researchers are fostering a more inclusive and diversified approach to patient care, acknowledging the potential benefits of plant-based interventions in preventing and managing chronic diseases.

OPPORTUNITIES AND DIFFICULTIES

Despite the promising advancements in plant-based medicine, challenges persist on the road to widespread integration into mainstream healthcare. Standardization of plant-derived products, quality control, and regulatory frameworks pose significant hurdles, as variations in plant composition can impact the consistency and efficacy of treatments. Additionally, the need for rigorous clinical trials and evidence-based research is paramount to validate the safety and effectiveness of plant-based therapies, ensuring their acceptance within the medical community.

Opportunities, however, abound in overcoming these challenges. Collaborative efforts between the pharmaceutical industry, academic institutions, and regulatory bodies can establish robust guidelines for the development and commercialization of plant-based medicines. Increased public awareness and acceptance of alternative therapies further create a conducive environment for the integration of plant-based medicine into healthcare systems. As the demand for natural and sustainable healthcare solutions continues to rise, the future holds the promise of more harmonious coexistence between traditional and plant-based medicinal practices, offering patients a diverse array of therapeutic options for enhanced well-being.